AORTIC ANEURYSM REPAIR DIET

Revitalizing Your Health And Understanding Dietary Solutions For Cardiovascular Recovery And Relief

DR LUCAS KAYCE

DISCLAIMER

This book about illness and nutrition is not meant to replace expert medical advice, diagnosis, or treatment; rather, it is meant purely for informational reasons. This book's content is founded on broad concepts and recommendations for managing diseases and nutrition.

Before adopting any major dietary or lifestyle changes, readers are recommended to speak with a qualified healthcare provider, such as a licensed physician or registered dietitian, especially if they have pre-existing medical concerns. Everybody has different health demands, so what works for one person might not work for another.

The use of the information provided in this book may have unfavorable repercussions or consequences, for which the author and publisher disclaim all liability. No disease is meant to be identified, treated, cured, or prevented by the information provided.

The book may include contain references to medical literature or research findings; however readers are urged to independently confirm this material and contact reliable sources.

It is important to remember that the fields of nutrition and medicine are always changing, and that new findings could have an impact on the advice offered in this book. As a result, readers are urged to keep up with the most recent advancements in healthcare and, when in doubt, seek professional counsel.

By reading this book, readers agree that they are in charge of their own health decisions and release the author and publisher from any liability arising from the use of the material in the book, whether direct or indirect.

TABLE OF CONTENTS

ABOUT THE BOOK

Aortic aneurysm repair is a crucial part of cardiovascular health, and the book "Aortic Aneurysm Repair Diet" highlights the role that dietary decisions play in supporting and controlling this condition. This book is significant because it offers a thorough examination of the connection between nutrition and the health of an aortic aneurysm, which can help those dealing with the difficulties associated with this medical condition.

The book's goal is introduced in the first section, which also emphasizes how important food is to the treatment and management of aortic aneurysms. The book makes sure that readers have a complete awareness of aortic aneurysms, including their types, causes, symptoms, and potential treatment options, with a particular focus on surgical repair, by going into great detail on the condition.

The relevance of nutrition in the comprehensive therapy of aortic aneurysms is further explained, which again emphasizes the complex relationship between dietary decisions and cardiovascular health. The dietary requirements covered, which includes information on important nutrients including antioxidants, omega-3 fatty acids, and necessary vitamins and minerals, are laid out in this chapter.

Practical advice on creating a diet that effectively repairs aortic aneurysms can be found. Comprehensive information on foods to limit or avoid reducing hazards is provided to readers, along with suggestions for meals to include for best vascular health. About developing a balanced meal plan, the book provides useful advice along with meal ideas and helpful cooking instructions.

The book addresses a wider range of lifestyle factors that impact the health of an aortic aneurysm, going beyond diet alone. Advocating for consistent exercise, stress reduction, and quitting smoking, it recognizes the need for a holistic approach to achieve overall well-being.

The continuing aspect of managing an aortic aneurysm is covered, which emphasizes the value of routine examinations and the necessity for people to pay attention to their bodies. It gives the book a useful edge by including a range of heart-healthy recipes that follow the previously mentioned dietary guidelines.

The "Aortic Aneurysm Repair Diet" is an invaluable tool for anyone looking to maximize their dietary decisions about aortic aneurysm repair. It provides a comprehensive and useful manual for improved cardiovascular health.

CHAPTER ONE

IMPORTANCE OF DIET FOR REPAIRING AORTIC ANEURYSMS

It is impossible to exaggerate the significance of nutrition in the context of aortic aneurysm repair because it is essential for both prevention and recuperation after surgery. Because aortic aneurysms can be fatal, a thorough understanding of the condition is necessary to treat its intricacies. Aortic aneurysms, which are defined as abnormal bulges in the aorta, the biggest artery in the body, can be of many forms, and each one requires therapy that takes specific factors into account.

KNOWING ABOUT AORTIC ANEURYSMS

It is essential to comprehend aortic aneurysms to fully appreciate how serious the situation is. If left untreated, these aberrant aortic expansions, which can develop in various arterial segments, might pose serious hazards. A thorough investigation into the description and varieties of aortic aneurysms reveals the complexities surrounding this medical issue and highlights the need for customized therapies.

REASONS AND DANGER ELEMENTS

Aortic aneurysm causes and risk factors help to clarify the complex nature of this vascular condition. A comprehensive approach to patient care is crucial since aortic aneurysms can arise as a result of lifestyle decisions, age, and genetics. By carefully analyzing these variables, it is possible to determine who is more likely to develop an aortic aneurysm and to take preventative and early intervention treatments.

SIGNS AND PROGNOSIS

Identifying the signs and using efficient diagnostic techniques are essential in the treatment of aortic aneurysms. These aneurysms are asymptomatic, which emphasizes the need for routine tests for early identification. When present, symptoms could include pulsations, discomfort, or other signs that demand medical care. Healthcare practitioners can precisely determine the size and severity of the aneurysm using diagnostic techniques including imaging investigations and physical exams, which helps to determine the best course of action.

OPTIONS FOR TREATMENT, INCLUDING SURGICAL REPAIR

A variety of procedures are available to address aortic aneurysms in terms of treatment, including surgical repair. The size, location, and general health of the patient are among the criteria that impact the choice to proceed with surgical treatment. Whether open or endovascular, surgery is a vital option for treating aortic aneurysms, to reduce the risk of rupture and avert potentially disastrous outcomes.

Among these factors, nutrition becomes a modifiable factor that can have a major effect on the results of aortic aneurysm repair.

Healthy eating habits can impact vascular function, which lays the groundwork for both preoperative planning and postoperative recuperation. In addition to surgical proficiency, a comprehensive approach to patient care must take into account the complex interactions between food and the dynamics of aortic aneurysms. This thorough investigation highlights the value of a multifaceted approach to patient care by laying the groundwork for a deeper comprehension of the interrelated factors that influence the treatment of aortic aneurysms.

CHAPTER TWO

DIETARY GUIDELINES FOR THE TREATMENT OF AORTIC ANEURYSMS

SUMMARY OF NUTRITION AND HEART HEALTH

One of the most important aspects of managing an aortic aneurysm is being aware of how nutrition affects cardiovascular health. Aortic aneurysms is one of the risk factors for cardiovascular illnesses that is significantly influenced by diet. Eating a diet high in nutrients that support healthy cardiovascular function and general well-being is what is commonly associated with a heart-healthy diet.

THE IMPACT OF DIET ON THE DEVELOPMENT AND PROGRESSION OF AORTIC ANEURYSMS

There is a complex association between nutrition and the onset and development of aortic aneurysms. Atherosclerosis and hypertension are two risk factors for aortic aneurysms that might be exacerbated by certain dietary choices.

Excessive consumption of cholesterol, trans fats, and saturated fats can exacerbate or cause the development of plaque in the arteries, weakening the aortic wall and increasing the risk of aneurysm formation or exacerbation.

Conversely, a diet high in vitamins, minerals, and antioxidants might be protective. Fruits and vegetables are rich in antioxidants, which can help fight oxidative stress, which is linked to the development of aneurysms. Furthermore, it's critical to keep a healthy weight through an appropriate diet, as obesity can exacerbate the illness by putting more strain on the blood vessels.

NUTRITIONAL NEEDS OF PATIENTS WITH AORTIC ANEURYSMS

Those who have been diagnosed with aortic aneurysms need to follow a particular set of dietary recommendations. The goals of these recommendations are to promote general cardiovascular health and control risk factors. The first and most important thing to do is to regulate blood pressure with diet.

This entails consuming less sodium because consuming too much salt might raise blood pressure. Bananas and leafy greens are two foods high in potassium that may help keep blood pressure in check.

Omega-3 fatty acids, which have anti-inflammatory qualities and are present in fatty fish like salmon and walnuts, are part of a diet aimed at enhancing artery health. Omega-3 fatty acids may lessen inflammation and increase vascular flexibility.

Furthermore, stressing the need for a diet that is well-balanced and rich in whole grains, lean proteins, fruits, and vegetables is crucial for acquiring a range of nutrients that are vital for cardiovascular health.

Healthcare providers should be consulted when creating customized eating plans, which should take the patient's general health, comorbidities, and prescription schedules into account.

A thorough strategy for managing an aortic aneurysm must include regular monitoring of nutritional status and dietary modifications as necessary.

A careful and customized dietary strategy can help manage risk factors and potentially decrease the course of aortic aneurysms, which is essential to the overall treatment and well-being of these patients.

CHAPTER THREE

CRUCIAL ELEMENTS FOR HEALING AORTIC ANEURYSM

ANTIOXIDANTS: WHAT THEY DO

By reducing oxidative stress and inflammation, antioxidants are essential for aortic aneurysm healing. Because it weakens the artery walls, oxidative stress plays a major role in the development of aortic aneurysms. Antioxidants, which include beta-carotene, selenium, and vitamins C and E, neutralize free radicals and lessen inflammation and oxidative damage. These substances aid in preserving the aorta's structural integrity and may impede the aneurysm's advancement.

HEALTH OF THE HEART AND OMEGA-3 FATTY ACIDS

Omega-3 fatty acids are vital for heart function and are important in the healing of aortic aneurysms. Omega-3 fatty acids, which are present in fatty fish like salmon and mackerel, have anti-inflammatory qualities that may lessen arterial wall inflammation. Additionally, they enhance blood vessel elasticity, lower triglyceride levels, and improve lipid profiles, all of which improve cardiovascular health overall.

For those with aortic aneurysms, including foods high in omega-3 fatty acids in their diet or taking supplements may be helpful as it may aid in the healing process and lower the chance of problems.

MINERALS AND VITAMINS FOR CARDIOVASCULAR HEALTH

Vitamins and minerals are vital for the health of blood vessels, particularly the aorta since they keep the blood vessels strong and flexible. For example, the manufacture of collagen, a protein that gives blood vessels structural support, depends on vitamin C.

The integrity of the artery walls is preserved by collagen, which keeps the walls from weakening and developing aneurysms.

Furthermore, vitamin K can help avoid excessive bleeding and is essential for good blood coagulation, both of which are important during surgical procedures to treat aortic aneurysms.

Minerals that are important for vascular health include magnesium and potassium. To keep the already compromised artery walls from being further stressed, potassium helps control blood pressure.

Magnesium, on the other hand, helps the blood vessels relax and supports muscle and nerve function. People who have aortic aneurysms may benefit from this relaxation effect since it lessens the likelihood of problems and lessens the burden on the heart.

Sustaining vascular health and promoting the healing of aortic aneurysms require a diet high in antioxidants, omega-3 fatty acids, vitamins, and minerals. Together, these nutrients help lower inflammation and oxidative stress while strengthening the structural integrity of blood arteries, particularly the aorta.

Although dietary interventions are beneficial, people with aortic aneurysms should speak with medical professionals for individualized guidance and management plans catered to their unique medical requirements.

CHAPTER FOUR

ITEMS TO ADD TO YOUR DIET TO HELP REPAIR AORTIC ANEURYSMS

PRODUCE AND FRUITS

Consuming a wide range of fruits and vegetables is essential for those having surgery to repair an aortic aneurysm. Essential vitamins, minerals, and antioxidants included in these nutrient-dense foods support cardiovascular health as a whole. Vitamins C and K, found in abundance in fruits like berries, citrus fruits, and apples, are important for the production of collagen and blood clotting, respectively. On the other hand, vegetables high in fiber, such as leafy greens, broccoli, and carrots, support healthy digestion and help with weight management.

The healing process following aortic aneurysm repair can be aided by the high antioxidant content found in fruits and vegetables, which can also help minimize oxidative stress and inflammation.

COMPLETE GRAINS

Another essential element of the diet for aortic aneurysm repair is whole grains. Eating foods high in fiber, complex carbs, and other nutrients—such as brown rice, quinoa, and whole wheat bread—helps maintain gut health and long-term energy. Magnesium and potassium, two elements necessary for sustaining blood pressure within a healthy range, are also found in whole grains. People can better control their blood sugar levels and lower their chance of complications during the recovery phase following aortic aneurysm repair by choosing whole grains versus refined grains.

TRIM PROTEINS

The post-aortic aneurysm repair diet must include lean proteins since they are vital to tissue preservation and repair. Lean protein sources include tofu, fish, lentils, and fowl. These foods high in protein supply the amino acids required for muscular growth and tissue repair. Additionally, by lowering inflammation and increasing blood vessel flexibility, consuming omega-3 fatty acids from fish like salmon or trout can benefit heart health. A varied food intake is ensured by keeping a balance between various protein sources, promoting general healing and well-being.

GOOD FATS

The aortic aneurysm repair diet must include healthy fats since they support cardiovascular health and general well-being. Olive oil, almonds, seeds, and avocados are good sources of healthful fats. Monounsaturated and polyunsaturated fatty acids, which are present in these fats, can lower cholesterol and lower the risk of cardiovascular problems. Flaxseeds and fatty fish, which are high in omega-3 fatty acids, have anti-inflammatory qualities that may speed up recovery and lessen the chance of problems after surgery. Moderate consumption of these heart-healthy fats contributes to a comprehensive and heart-healthy strategy for the repair and rehabilitation of aortic aneurysms.

Patients having aortic aneurysm repair must eat a diet rich in nutrients and balance. Whole grains provide complex carbs and important minerals, while fruits and vegetables provide vital vitamins and antioxidants. Healthy fats are essential for fostering cardiovascular health, while lean proteins support muscle growth and tissue repair. Following aortic aneurysm repair, people can promote their recuperation and improve their general well-being by including these food groups in their diet.

CHAPTER FIVE

THE EFFECT OF SODIUM ON BLOOD PRESSURE

Sodium, which is frequently present in salt, is essential for preserving the fluid balance in the body and supporting neuronal activity. On the other hand, consuming too much salt is associated with hypertension, a significant risk factor for cardiovascular illnesses. Elevated sodium levels cause the body to hold onto more water to counteract the concentration, which raises blood pressure and increases blood volume. Limiting sodium consumption is crucial to reducing the risk of hypertension and the health issues that come with it.

TRANS FATS AND SATURATED FATS

Dietary fats that are high in trans and saturated fats can lead to several health problems. Animal goods including red meat, butter, and full-fat dairy products are major sources of saturated fats, which are solid at room temperature. Contrarily, trans fats are produced artificially through a procedure known as hydrogenation and are frequently found in processed meals and baked goods that are sold commercially. The risk of heart disease and stroke can be increased by consuming any type of fat or by raising LDL cholesterol levels. It is essential to limit the intake of foods high in trans and saturated fats to preserve heart health.

ALCOHOL AND CAFFEINE

Coffee, tea, energy drinks, and some pharmaceuticals all include caffeine, a stimulant of the central nervous system that can have both beneficial and detrimental effects on health. While moderate caffeine consumption may have positive effects including increased alertness and cognitive performance, excessive caffeine use might have unfavorable effects.

Excessive amounts of caffeine can elevate heart rate, induce jitters, and cause insomnia.

Moreover, different people react differently to caffeine in terms of blood pressure; some may experience a brief increase. Caffeine use should be kept to a minimum, especially for people who are already experiencing cardiovascular problems or are sensitive to its effects.

Moderate alcohol use may provide certain health advantages, especially for heart health. On the other hand, excessive and prolonged alcohol consumption can cause several health complications, including heart problems, liver disease, and a higher risk of developing several types of cancer.

Because alcohol affects the nervous system and throws off the balance between sympathetic and parasympathetic processes, it directly affects blood pressure. Reducing alcohol consumption is crucial to preserving general health and lowering the likelihood of related problems.

Making educated dietary decisions requires knowledge of how the body reacts to alcohol, caffeine, saturated and trans fats, and sodium.

People can greatly aid in preserving their best health and averting the emergence of many diseases, especially those linked to cardiovascular health, by consuming these substances in moderation.

CHAPTER SIX

DEVELOPING A BALANCED MEAL PLAN FOR AORTIC ANEURYSM REPAIR

DIETARY GUIDELINES IN GENERAL

For patients having aortic aneurysm repair, a balanced meal plan should be prepared according to basic dietary standards that support the healing process and overall cardiovascular health. Maintaining optimal healing and minimizing risk factors require a heart-healthy diet. It is crucial to stress the importance of eating a diet high in fruits, vegetables, whole grains, lean meats, and healthy fats. These nutrient-dense meals support the general health of the cardiovascular system by offering vital vitamins, minerals, antioxidants, and fiber.

Reducing the consumption of trans and saturated fats is essential for controlling cholesterol levels and avoiding issues throughout the healing process. Furthermore, since too much salt can cause fluid retention and put stress on the cardiovascular system, controlling sodium consumption is essential to sustaining appropriate blood pressure levels. Eating foods high in omega-3 fatty acids, such as walnuts, flaxseeds, and fatty fish, can reduce inflammation and promote heart health.

EXAMPLE MENUS

To support healing and general cardiovascular health, patients recovering from aortic aneurysm repair should follow a well-balanced diet that includes a range of nutrient-rich foods. A heart-healthy breakfast of whole-grain oatmeal with fresh berries and a few nuts for extra fiber and heart-healthy lipids might be the beginning of a normal day. A tiny portion of Greek yogurt topped with chia seeds or sliced veggies with hummus would make tasty snacks.

Lean protein sources, such as grilled chicken, fish, or lentils, should be the main course of lunch and dinner. They should be served with colorful vegetables and nutritious grains, like brown rice or quinoa. A range of veggies contributes to taste and texture while also offering vital vitamins and antioxidants.

You can cook with or add healthy fats to salads from sources like avocado or olive oil. Controlling portion sizes is essential for avoiding overindulgence and maintaining a healthy weight, both of which are good for cardiovascular health.

A handful of almonds, some fresh fruit, or whole-grain crackers paired with low-fat cheese are some examples of between-meal snacks. Water, herbal teas, or water flavored with cucumber or citrus slices are great sources of hydration, which is also crucial for general health.

ADVICE ON COOKING AND MEAL PREPARATION

A balanced meal plan for aortic aneurysm repair can be greatly enhanced by using effective cooking and meal preparation techniques. Selecting cooking techniques like baking, grilling, steaming, or sautéing in place of frying might aid in lowering the total fat level of meals. Enhancing the flavor of food without endangering heart health can be achieved by seasoning it with herbs, spices, and citrus instead of using too much salt.

Time can be saved and nutrient-dense selections can be guaranteed when meals are prepared ahead of time. Lean protein, whole grain, and roasted veggie batches make it easy to quickly put together well-balanced meals every day of the week. To guarantee that each meal has a wide range of nutrients, it's critical to concentrate on adding a diversity of colors and textures.

When shopping for groceries, give priority to nutritious grains, lean meats, and fresh produce over processed and high-sodium foods. Making educated decisions can be facilitated by reading food labels, particularly when it comes to added sugars and hidden sources of harmful fats. Furthermore, seeking advice from a qualified nutritionist or healthcare provider can offer tailored recommendations based on dietary choices and unique health requirements.

CHAPTER SEVEN

HYDRATION: ITS SIGNIFICANCE

WATER'S SIGNIFICANCE FOR CARDIOVASCULAR HEALTH

Water is vital for several physiological processes in the body, including the maintenance of cardiovascular health. Sufficient fluid intake is closely related to the heart's ability to operate as it should. Maintaining blood volume is one of water's fundamental roles, which helps to maintain ideal blood pressure levels. Dehydration can cause the blood volume to drop, which may put more strain on the heart and raise blood pressure.

Moreover, enough hydration promotes the body's ability to transfer oxygen and nutrients throughout, which help the cardiovascular system operate as efficiently as possible. Water is necessary for blood viscosity, which makes blood flow easily through blood vessels and lowers the chance of clot formation.

Dehydration may lead to thicker blood, which increases the risk of cardiovascular problems and makes the heart work harder to pump blood.

SUGGESTED FLUID CONSUMPTION

Several variables, such as age, sex, degree of physical activity, and weather, affect the required fluid intake. But generally speaking, it's recommended to drink eight 8-ounce glasses of water or more each day—a practice known as the "8x8 rule." This is roughly equivalent to two liters or half a gallon. It is important to remember that each person may have different demands for hydration and that changes should be made according to things like the level of exercise, the outside temperature, and general health.

The ideal fluid intake is also influenced by variables like weight and age. For example, the aging process can impair an individual's body's ability to detect thirst, thus older folks may need to be especially careful about staying hydrated.

In a similar vein, people who exercise vigorously might need to drink more water to replace the fluids they lose through perspiration.

DRINKS TO SELECT AND STEER CLEAR OF

Making the correct beverage choices is essential for sustaining appropriate hydration levels and advancing general health. The best, most natural way to stay hydrated is with water, which has no calories. Herbal teas and infused water are also healthy substitutes that help you stay hydrated without adding calories or sweets.

Conversely, some drinks ought to be avoided entirely or only taken in moderation. Sugary beverages, like sodas and fruit juices with added sugar, can raise calorie consumption too much, which can result in weight gain and other cardiovascular problems. Coffee and tea are examples of caffeinated beverages that can help you stay hydrated, but you should only take them in moderation as too much caffeine can have diuretic effects.

Maintaining optimal hydration and general well-being requires knowledge of the function that water plays in cardiovascular health, adherence to suggested fluid intake guidelines, and making wise beverage consumption decisions. Maintaining a regular and sufficient level of hydration is essential to leading a healthy lifestyle, as it aids in the correct operation of the cardiovascular system and supports other physiological functions in the body.

CHAPTER EIGHT

AORTIC ANEURYSM HEALTH THROUGH LIFESTYLE MODIFICATIONS

FREQUENT EXERCISE AND ITS ADVANTAGES FOR THE HEART

Frequent exercise is essential for maintaining cardiovascular health, and it becomes even more critical for those who have aortic aneurysms. Regular physical activity strengthens the cardiac muscles, improves blood circulation, and helps people become more cardiovascularly fit overall. Keeping the circulatory system in good condition is crucial for aortic aneurysm patients to lower their risk of problems. To make sure an exercise program is safe and appropriate for a person's health, it is necessary to speak with medical professionals before beginning one.

Regular exercise has more benefits for the cardiovascular system than just its immediate effects on the heart. Being physically active helps people control their weight, which is important for those who have aortic aneurysms because being overweight can put stress on the heart? Moreover, exercise promotes a healthy cardiovascular profile by assisting in the regulation of blood pressure, cholesterol, and blood sugar. A balanced, moderate exercise regimen, such as swimming, cycling, or brisk walking, can make a big difference in the quality of life for people who have aortic aneurysms.

TECHNIQUES FOR STRESS MANAGEMENT

Techniques for managing stress are essential for the general health and well-being of those who have aortic aneurysms. Prolonged stress can lead to higher heart rate and blood pressure, which further strains the already fragile walls of an aortic aneurysm. Stress-reduction techniques like yoga, deep breathing exercises, and mindfulness meditation can be incorporated to assist in controlling stress levels and fostering calmness. Smoking Cessation and its Effect on Aortic Aneurysms: This could therefore have a beneficial effect on the cardiovascular system and possibly lower the risk of complications related to aortic aneurysms.

For those who have aortic aneurysms, quitting smoking is essential because of the negative impact smoking has on cardiovascular health. In addition to raising heart rate and blood pressure, smoking also adds to the accumulation of plaque in the arteries, which weakens the blood vessels. Tobacco products contain compounds that can weaken the aortic walls, increasing a person's risk of aneurysm formation and rupture. One of the most effective ways to enhance cardiovascular health and slow the development of aortic aneurysms is to give up smoking. To increase the likelihood of successfully stopping, it is advised to look for assistance from medical professionals or programs that help people stop smoking.

Modifying one's lifestyle is essential to controlling and enhancing the health of those who have aortic aneurysms. When done carefully, regular exercise improves cardiovascular health and general well-being.

The cardiovascular system is negatively impacted by prolonged stress, however, stress management strategies can lessen this effect. Additionally, quitting smoking is essential to halting further deterioration of the compromised blood vessels. When combined with routine medical monitoring, these lifestyle modifications can greatly improve the quality of life for those who have aortic aneurysms.

CHAPTER NINE

FREQUENT EVALUATIONS AND SUGGESTIONS

Patients who have had aortic aneurysm repair should be closely monitored and have their diets adjusted regularly. These regular check-ups with medical specialists aid in monitoring the patient's general health, evaluating the efficacy of the medication, and spotting any possible side effects. Healthcare professionals can keep a close eye on things like blood pressure, cholesterol, and the patient's general cardiovascular health during these examinations. They can also offer insightful information on dietary changes that could be required to promote recovery and avert more issues.

PAYING ATTENTION TO YOUR BODY

After aortic aneurysm repair, it's critical to pay attention to your body's needs when it comes to eating. Patients should be aware of how their bodies react to various foods and nutritional options. This includes being aware of any discomfort, fluctuations in energy, or potential digestive problems. People who are aware of these signals can make educated dietary choices by avoiding meals that could increase risks or difficulties and identifying foods that have a beneficial impact on their well-being. Optimal recovery and long-term health depend on a customized nutrition plan based on each person's unique demands and responses.

BRINGING ABOUT LONG-TERM CHANGES

A vital part of the rehabilitation process after aortic aneurysm treatment is implementing long-lasting dietary adjustments. People are recommended to concentrate on developing a balanced and sustainable dietary plan that supports general cardiovascular health rather than implementing drastic or temporary interventions. This entails including a range of foods high in nutrients, including whole grains, fruits, vegetables, lean meats, and healthy fats. Creating long-term routines that enhance cardiovascular health and general well-being, such as regular exercise and stress reduction, are other examples of sustainable adjustments. To make sure that dietary modifications are reasonable and long-term sustainable, consistency and little alterations are stressed.

Following aortic aneurysm repair, diet monitoring, and alterations require a comprehensive strategy that incorporates routine examinations, careful attention to physiological cues, and the execution of long-term dietary modifications. These tactics seek to enhance cardiovascular health, maximize recuperation, and avert any problems. Individuals who have undergone aortic aneurysm repair will benefit from improved overall well-being and long-term health if they work closely with healthcare experts and make informed tailored decisions.

CHAPTER TEN

RECIPES FOR HEART-HEALTHY

BREAKFASTS AND AORTIC ANEURYSM REPAIR

Repairing an aortic aneurysm is an important medical treatment, and recovery from the surgery depends greatly on the post-operative diet. Keeping up a heart-healthy diet is one of the most important things to think about, beginning with breakfast choices. Choosing whole grains can give you a decent supply of fiber and other important nutrients. Examples of whole grains are oatmeal and whole wheat bread. Fruits like bananas and berries provide natural sweetness and essential vitamins.

It is advised to have lean proteins for breakfast in addition to nutritious grains and fruits. Without being overly saturated in fat, eggs—especially egg whites—can be a fantastic source of protein. Think about including heart-healthy fats from foods like almonds and avocados, which are rich in omega-3 fatty acids and improve cardiovascular health in general. These breakfast options promote the healing process following aortic aneurysm repair by providing a nutritious and well-balanced start to the day.

LUNCH IDEAS HIGH IN NUTRIENTS

Creating nutrient-dense lunch ideas is essential for those undergoing aortic aneurysm repair recovery. Vitamins and minerals can be obtained by emphasizing a range of vibrant vegetables in salads or as side dishes. For example, foods high in leafy greens, bell peppers, and tomatoes support heart health. Lean proteins like chicken or fish that have been baked or grilled can be incorporated to guarantee a sufficient protein intake without endangering cardiovascular health.

Complex carbs, such as those found in whole grains like brown rice and quinoa, provide energy without sharp rises in blood sugar levels. Dressings made with heart-healthy oils, such as olive oil, provide flavor and heart-healthy monounsaturated fats. Lunch alternatives high in nutrients are a great way for people to provide their bodies with the fuel they need for recuperation and general health.

HEALTHY RECIPES FOR DINNER

Healthy supper recipes are an essential component of the dietary plan for post-aortic aneurysm repair since they support healing and maintain health. Choosing lean protein sources, like fish, tofu, or grilled fowl, guarantees that you're getting enough protein for your body to heal and repair your muscles. Incorporating an array of vibrant veggies into stir-fries or roasting meals enriches the diet with vital vitamins, minerals, and fiber.

Adding nutritious grains to dinner meals, such as quinoa or whole wheat pasta, helps to maintain cardiovascular health and gives you lasting energy. Restricting salt consumption is essential because too much sodium can cause hypertension, which is a risk after aortic aneurysm repair. Enhancing food flavor without sacrificing health objectives is possible when fresh herbs and spices are used as flavorings instead of salt.

An approach to post-surgery eating that is comprehensive and nourishing involves the use of healthy meal recipes.

SNACKS AND DESSERTS

Choosing the right snacks and desserts is crucial for patients recovering from aortic aneurysm repair because it can be difficult to eat heart-healthy during these times. Nutrient-dense snacks, such as a piece of fruit or a handful of almonds, offer a filling and healthful alternative. Another great option is Greek yogurt with berries, which provides antioxidants, probiotics, and protein.

Moderation is essential when it comes to sweets. Think about including healthy dessert alternatives, including fruit-based dishes or ones with whole grains and natural sweeteners. Because of its high antioxidant content, dark chocolate can be a heart-healthy option when consumed in moderation.